# Advocate
## for Your
# Health

# Advocate
## for Your
# Health

## A STEP-BY-STEP GUIDE TO
## NAVIGATING MEDICAL VISITS

### Henraya F. McGruder, PhD
CEO, Audacious Health Advocates, LLC

MYND
MATTERS

To purchase books in bulk or for additional information, contact the publisher.

Published by Mynd Matters Publishing
2690 Cobb Parkway SE
Ste A5-375
Smyrna, GA 30080
www.myndmatterspublishing.com

ISBN: 978-1-963874-62-4


FIRST EDITION

# Disclaimer

*Advocate for Your Health* was conceived to be useful for individuals who are disproportionately more likely to have chronic diseases in the United States. Those individuals are typically people who are from racially and ethnically diverse populations. However, the information contained in these pages is not only useful for those populations but also for all individuals, regardless of race and/or ethnicity.

The content focuses on the patient when engaged in the healthcare setting and provides tips on how to self-advocate and make the most out of any medical visit. I hope individuals become an integral part of *their own* healthcare team.

While this book does not focus on other aspects of healthcare, such as navigating insurance or governmental coverage (e.g., Medicaid and Medicare), I hope that learning how to effectively self-advocate will become a common practice not only in the broader healthcare space but in all aspects of life.

# Contents

# Preface

The idea for this book originated from my career in public health at the federal level. I began working at the Centers for Disease Control and Prevention (CDC) in 2002 as an epidemiologist, a professional who studies diseases and how they are identified, transmitted, and controlled within populations. My assignment was to work on issues related to cardiovascular diseases and stroke.

In my role, I published several articles highlighting the differences between population groups related to heart attack and stroke occurrence. I also examined the differences between population groups around the risk factors that lead to the development of heart disease and stroke. The results typically showed that the population groups most affected by high rates of disease and more risk factors were people of color, often African Americans and Hispanics. I noticed that this finding was not just in my research but also in other published manuscripts. In the research, the differences between groups were highlighted, but less was mentioned about what individuals could do during medical visits to reduce the risks of developing diseases or prevent death from these diseases. These results and findings disturbed me and I wanted so badly to do something to change this in some way. Wanting to reduce the diseases and death rates among groups of people is addressing a health disparity (a particular type of health difference that is closely linked with social, economic, and/or environmental disadvantage (Healthy People 2020).

"Health disparities adversely affect groups of people who have systematically experienced greater obstacles to health based on their racial or ethnic group; religion; socioeconomic status; gender; age; mental health; cognitive, sensory, or physical disability; sexual orientation or gender identity; geographic location; or other characteristics historically linked to racism, discrimination, or exclusion." (Healthy People 2020)

As a result of my research and interests, I ultimately discovered that my passion was to examine ideas and avenues to reduce and/or eliminate health disparities. When I retired from CDC after twenty years of public service, Audacious Health Advocates, LLC was born. The organization aims to provide people with the education they need to advocate for themselves in the healthcare space, to feel empowered to ask questions to help them partner with their physicians, and to ultimately improve risk factors, diseases, and conditions that disproportionately affect minority populations, thereby reducing health disparities. This was my way to address health disparities—my true passion. There is no better time to share this information and change the direction of our health in a positive way.

"I learned a long time ago the wisest thing I can do is be on my own side, be an advocate for myself and others like me."

—Maya Angelou

# The Science

As a former employee of the U.S. Government, I published articles that describe the occurrence of diseases and conditions among American adults. The data on Americans is often collected through national surveys that ask demographic questions (e.g., age, sex, marital status) as well as many questions about health conditions, diseases, and current health behaviors. Epidemiologists are typically tasked with interpreting the survey results and informing the public via manuscripts and publications. Often, the media highlights the results of these published studies on local and national news outlets and media websites.

The average person may never come across the published studies but will pay attention to the short news reports in the media, such as radio, television, the internet, and social media. Because this information can be intimidating to read in its longer form, the comprehensive results and detailed findings are not widely known. For example, many studies compare demographic variables in relation to a specific disease/condition. Often, the results show differences among groups based on age, race, sex, and other factors. More specifically, the results will indicate that certain groups have a higher prevalence of medical conditions compared to other groups. For example, there are significant racial/ethnic differences in pregnancy care, with non-Hispanic Black women incurring three to four times higher rates of pregnancy-related death compared to non-Hispanic white women (Collier and Molina, 2019). The racial/ethnic differences related to maternal mortality were even highlighted as a White House initiative in 2022 entitled Blueprint for Addressing the Maternal Health Crisis.[1] The need to bring national attention to this issue was due to the health disparity experienced by groups of women belonging to particular racial/ethnic groups, like Black women, native women, and women living in rural communities.

Another example of racial/ethnic health disparities can be observed in stroke. According to the

---

[1] https://bidenwhitehouse.archives.gov/briefing-room/statements-releases/2024/07/10/the-white-house-blueprint-for-addressing-the-maternal-health-crisis-two-years-of-progress/; accessed March 11, 2025

Mayo Clinic, stroke is a medical emergency that occurs when the blood supply to part of the brain is blocked or reduced.[2] According to the CDC, non-Hispanic Black adults and Pacific Islander adults have the highest rates of death from stroke compared to other groups. Additionally, the risk of having a first stroke is nearly twice as high for non-Hispanic Blacks compared to non-Hispanic White adults.[3] These findings highlight another example of health disparities experienced between population groups.

Many takeaways of recommendations from these studies will provide blanket suggestions to state programs on how to reduce the occurrence of diseases and conditions. While I have only highlighted two examples, numerous studies conducted over decades have also revealed these health disparities. My goal is to encourage individuals to take a more active role in their own medical care, helping to turn these health trends in a healthier direction.

---

[2] https://www.mayoclinic.org/diseases-conditions/stroke/symptoms-causes/syc-20350113; accessed March 11, 2025

[3] https://www.cdc.gov/stroke/data-research/facts-stats/ Accessed March 11, 2025

In a research study, more than half of adults stated they use the internet to research medical information.[4] According to this study, respondents searched for the following information: nutrition or diet information, drug side effects or complications of medical therapy, or alternative medicine. In 2023, research showed women were more likely to use the internet or search engines to look for health or medical information compared to men.[5] Additionally, the percentage of adults using the internet to access health or medical information was higher among White and Asian adults compared to other groups. Of note, education levels were not compared to see if those with higher levels of education use the internet to access health or medical information compared to those with lower levels of education.[6]

I have observed that most people (including me) search via Google to investigate symptoms and potentially diagnose themselves when they are having a health challenge. When browsing the internet for

---

[4] Diaz et al., 2002
[5] Wang and Cohen, 2023
[6] Wang and Cohen, 2023

results, individuals tend to find that the symptoms can range from mild conditions to "call 9-1-1 immediately." Most health care professionals will warn patients against using search engines to diagnose themselves. The gold standard is to seek the counsel of a medical professional instead. Please be advised that the internet and search engines are intended for informational purposes only and should not be used for medical diagnosis.

As health information technology has advanced over time, many health systems have implemented messaging tools that allow patients to send questions about their symptoms to healthcare professionals through a web-based portal. Healthcare professionals can advise you whether you need to be seen or if a condition can be handled at home with over-the-counter medications. These portals can also share medical test results with you instead of having to visit the doctor in person to receive these results. Ultimately, the internet and portals can be helpful or beneficial tools when combined with information from your medical professional. They can save time and provide avenues for direct communication when experiencing a health challenge, thereby alleviating the need to rely solely on the internet.

When choosing to use the internet to research health conditions, I recommend using reputable websites after obtaining a diagnosis from your healthcare professional. Websites such as CDC (www.cdc.gov) or the National Institutes of Health (NIH) (www.nih.gov) are valuable resources to visit for reliable and verified information concerning a diagnosis. The CDC and NIH are mandated to post information on their websites in plain language, which makes it easier to read, understand, and use government communications (www.plainlanguage.gov).

Efforts are being made to translate data from research studies into more accessible information for the general public. However, using websites and search engines to look for information on health conditions is typically the go-to for most Americans. I suggest using the reputable websites listed above to educate yourself on the diagnoses you get from your healthcare professional. However, please wait to search until *after* your medical appointment and a diagnosis has been made. If you have additional questions, please call or use the web-based portal to communicate directly with your healthcare team.

# The Goal of Advocacy

It can be intimidating to remember your medications, keep track of medical appointments, and understand the information shared during medical visits. The goal of health advocacy is to support you in the healthcare space, enabling you to increase your understanding and participation in your own healing and care. Another goal is to ease the burden and destigmatize fear of the healthcare space that some people may feel.

It is crucial for you to understand your disease/condition, be in tune with your symptoms, and how your body reacts to situations when symptoms worsen. This will enable you to feel confident in interacting with healthcare professionals and asking questions for a better understanding. If these steps are followed, you will be more actively engaged in your healing process.

More broadly, self-advocacy may positively affect diseases and conditions among populations with a higher level of disease prevalence. Being your own health advocate can help you live a healthier and longer life compared to those who leave health decisions to others without their participation. An example of a patient not advocating for themselves is when patients interact with doctors and do not ask questions, don't provide contextual information that is useful in their care, and let doctors make a care plan without their input. Interacting in this manner leaves a gap in the care continuum for the patient and can be easily remedied.

Trusted family members and friends can also act as health advocates for you and can be included in your healthcare team. If friends and family members are included on the team, they may participate in doctor visits and other health consultations to provide an additional ear in understanding the diagnosis of the disease/condition. As long as there is understanding of the diagnosis, a willingness to interact and ask questions of the health care professionals, then health advocacy is effective for the patient, regardless of who performs the task.

Health advocacy can begin at any age. It is ideal to start this practice as a child or adolescent, but it is essential at any age. According to an article at Weill

Cornell Medicine,[7] adolescence is a great age for patients to start advocating for their own health. Usually, parents are dismissed for a portion of medical visits with adolescents for them to be able to talk openly and honestly with the health care professionals without judgment from parents or guardians. If adolescents can form a trusting relationship with their health care team, they are more likely to adopt the suggestions from the visit and lead healthier lives. It is a great time to see themselves as part of the health care team, not just receiving care. They, indeed, do have a voice in their own care, and they can begin advocating for themselves in medical situations. Teens should ask questions during medical visits so they can seek a greater understanding, know their voice matters, and recognize that they are an essential part of their healthcare journey.

We have discussed why health advocacy is needed, highlighted and defined health disparities, and listed typical ways individuals address health concerns. Now, we will discuss how you can become more

---

[7] https://weillcornell.org/news/empowering-teens-to-be-their-own-health-advocates

involved in our own care and healing—essentially, how to self-advocate. I will outline five steps to help you become more involved, engage with a healthcare team, and ultimately change the trajectory of your health for the future.

Before we get into the "meat" of how you advocate for yourself, you must first understand the most important part of this effort. Many people believe that a doctor/healthcare professional is the expert in a medical situation. While they have a professional degree and a history of practicing medicine, they are never the expert on YOU. **You are the expert on you.** You know yourself better than anyone, so you should be able to advise the doctor about what will work best for you. Sometimes, the suggestions you will receive may not work for you and your lifestyle. If this is the case, only you can advocate and negotiate the terms of your care. You must consider yourself the expert on you and then work as a team with the professionals. Once this positioning is corrected in your mind, you will begin this journey in a new, more positive, and perhaps even more successful way. Remember, no one can tell you about yourself and what you are feeling better than you.

# Listen to Your Body

Most days, we go through life on autopilot. We have a routine that we follow every day, and we don't typically notice many changes or peculiarities. However, it is vital to pay attention to our bodies regularly and when we are experiencing a health challenge. Symptoms are the only way our bodies recognize that something is wrong, and we may need medical help. For example, does your body act differently when you eat a specific type of food? If you experience headaches frequently, do you notice any similar conditions, foods, or smells that occur at the same time? What about stomach pains? Do they occur after you eat specific things or exercise? Do your symptoms occur with some frequency, are they sudden, and what is the level of intensity?

Answers to these questions can lead you to helpful information about your body and provide valuable insights for a medical professional should you decide to seek medical help. When we don't pay attention to our bodies and symptoms, we are not able to provide as much insight to medical professionals as we can when we have been paying attention.

There are several bodily symptoms where immediate medical attention is required. If you experience shortness of breath, chest pains, and/or suddenly lose the ability to speak, walk, or talk, call 9-1-1 immediately. *It is important to note that the focus of this book is on less severe symptoms.*

Many healthcare professionals suggest patients keep symptom diaries to help diagnose a condition.[8] Symptom diaries are a simple and organized way to log or track your symptoms as they occur, allowing you to review them with a healthcare professional. The diaries are helpful as they can save time as the doctor doesn't have to ask as many questions, the notes become a part of the medical chart, the patient is more engaged in their own care, and it is free. A symptom diary can consist of the following categories: date, symptom, time, duration, intensity (1-10), triggers, treatment used, and

---

[8] *Hodge, 2013*

response. You can complete this symptom diary and provide it during your medical visit. Alternatively, a simple spreadsheet can capture this information well and can be submitted electronically to your healthcare professional through the web-based portal.

Here are some practical ways to learn to listen to your body. Make sure you get proper and restorative rest. According to the CDC, good sleep is essential for our health and emotional well-being. Being able to understand any message your body may be sending you is much easier when you are well-rested. If you are sleep deprived, you are less likely to notice these messages and gather this very important data.

Additionally, make sure you are honest when reporting symptoms and personal health information. If you choose to record your symptoms in a diary, be sure to be honest about when the symptoms occur and what they are. If you are not truthful about this information, you will not be able to receive accurate medical advice that can lead to the resolution of symptoms. Lastly, be curious. Curiosity helps you ask additional questions that may prompt you to want to learn more about what your body is doing.

# Know Your Family Health History

According to the CDC, knowing your family's health history can reduce your personal risk of disease and potentially change family health patterns for generations. While we cannot modify the existence of our family health history, it is a helpful tool in the toolbox to modify our own behaviors for an improved health outcome, but only if we act on the information we obtain.

The United States Surgeon General has designated Thanksgiving Day as National Family History Day to help families learn and collect information about their family health history. Collecting family health history reduces surprises and allows us to find out about diseases where we may be at higher risk, like heart disease, high blood pressure, glaucoma, cancer (breast, prostate, colorectal, etc.), depression, and/or diabetes. Collecting family history is low to no-cost, allows families to engage in meaningful and informative conversations that are helpful to many, and helps people understand the far-reaching effects of genetics.

The US Surgeon General's office has created a free, web-based tool to record this information called My Family Health Portrait.[9] Examples of family health history collection forms can be found in the reference links at the back of this book. Collecting family health history is not a one-time task. It is dynamic and should be updated when families evolve, as necessary. According to research, knowledge of family health history is low in the United States. While the majority of adults believe collecting this information is important, only 30% actively collected family health history in 2004. In a more recent study, 37% of surveyed adults had "a lot" of knowledge about family health history, while 60% reported knowing "some" family health history.[10]

---

[9] https://cbiit.github.io/FHH/html/index.html
[10] Hull and Natarajan, 2022

While collecting family health history is essential, it may not be easy to collect for various reasons. For example, it may evoke sad feelings about deceased family members, or family members may not want to engage in these conversations or may not recall any helpful information. However, it is still important to learn what you can and be sensitive to your family members during the process of collecting this truly valuable information. Remember, this information is not only helpful to you, it is useful to everyone in your family for generations to come.

Collecting family health history is vital, but it is also essential to share the information with your medical professionals. It should become a part of your official medical record. This information can help the doctor determine which types of screening tests or other interventions you may need and schedule them at the appropriate times. Even if the data you collect is not complete, any information you can share with a medical provider is helpful in your care.

When you are ready to collect your family health history, write down the names of your close blood relatives for both the maternal and paternal sides of your family, including parents, siblings, half-siblings, grandparents, aunts, uncles, nieces, and nephews. Ask them what medical conditions they have/have had and at what age they were first diagnosed. You may think you know this information, but be sure to confirm with the person.

Some diseases you may want to ask about are diabetes, high blood pressure (hypertension), high cholesterol, cancer, and stroke. You also may want to inquire about mental health conditions, such as depression, anxiety, or neurodivergent conditions, such as attention deficit hyperactivity disorder (ADHD) or autism. Feel free to use the "My Family Health Portrait" tool or search the internet for a table or spreadsheet to gather and record this information. It may be helpful to use a tool that allows the history to be shared electronically with other family members and medical professionals with ease. Remember, this information will not only help you but your family members as well.

Please note that the information you learn from collecting your family health history does not mean you will develop the disease/condition. However, being aware of your family history can help you take steps to reduce your risk of developing a condition. Your family health history cannot be modified, but you can change unhealthy behaviors by creating healthier habits to influence your health trajectory. For example, incorporating better eating habits and nutrition, increasing physical activity levels, and reducing smoking are ways to improve your own health regardless of your family's health history.

# Prepare for the Medical Visit

Now that we have learned about the science, about why advocating for yourself in the healthcare space is important, and know the importance of listening to your body and uncovering your family health history, you are now prepared to have a visit with your healthcare provider with an energized spirit.

The first thing you should do before a medical appointment is prepare. Prepare by documenting your symptoms using a symptom diary so you can speak about them with ease to the healthcare professional you will encounter during the visit. Many times, you will be asked about this more than once during the visit. The goal of describing your symptoms clearly is so the doctor can understand, try to identify the issue, and begin to resolve it. The way in which you describe your symptoms serves as a road map for the doctor. Symptoms may include changes in sleep patterns, pain in a certain area, an unexplained rash or bump, fever, or unexplained weight loss or gain. Be sure you can recall when the symptoms started, how long they have been occurring, and if they are getting better or worse.

Also, let them know if you have taken any medications to alleviate the symptoms. When discussing medications with your doctor, bring a list of all the daily medications, vitamins, and supplements you are currently taking. Medications that treat hypertension, cholesterol, cancer, or diabetes, and their dosages, are crucial during your conversation with the doctor. An example of a list where you can record all your medications, supplements, and vitamins can be found in the References & Resources section at the back of this book. Some medications interact with each other, and it is helpful for the doctor to have this information to best treat your disease/condition.

Many people struggle to remember the names and dosages of their medications, so it may be helpful to have them written down or take pictures of the bottle labels to present for the visit. If you attend a physician group (a group of doctors that participate in a practice), your medications and medical records may already be in one place (typically referred to as the electronic health record (EHR)), and accessing this information will be no issue.

Lastly, and almost most importantly, if you have an allergy to any medications, let the doctor know right away. If this information is not taken into consideration, you may have a severe reaction that could require immediate medical attention. Several resources in the References & Resources section will help you with your medications, thinking through crucial questions to ask the doctor, and tracking symptoms to assist you as you prepare for your appointment.

One last thing to remember is to be prepared to discuss your lifestyle habits. While patients are often asked about eating habits, physical activity levels, and sleep patterns, you should also be ready to talk about substance use, like alcohol intake, whether you smoke or vape, or use recreational drugs.[11] Your honesty is crucial here. Withholding this information may

---

[11] https://www.addictioncenter.com/community/honest-substance-use-doctor/

impede your progress on your health journey. If you genuinely care about getting better, don't worry about any judgment you may receive. Research shows that 82% of adults did not want to be judged or lectured about their substance use by their physician, while 61% of adults said they were embarrassed by their substance use. Reasons that you may be reluctant to discuss this information with your provider could be that you do not want this information to be part of your medical record, or you are not truly being honest with yourself about your substance use to be able to admit it. Either way, not disclosing this information can significantly impede your health journey.

# Speak Up and Ask Questions at The Medical Visit and Beyond

After you have prepared for your visit to the doctor, it is time to put the steps into action. With your symptom list, current medication list, and questions in hand, you are ready to start your medical visit. According to the Agency for Healthcare Research and Quality, the flow of the primary care medical visit is as follows:

*Step 1: Patient arrives at the office*

*Step 2: Office staff checks the patient in and checks to see if the patient has information in the EHR*

*Step 3: Patient is escorted to the exam room*

*Step 4: Medical assistant assesses vital signs (e.g., temperature, respiratory rate, oxygen saturation, and blood pressure)*

*Step 5: Healthcare professional reviews the vital signs and makes a clinical assessment*

*Step 6: Healthcare provider orders outpatient treatment regimen*

There are several points during this typical primary care visit where the patient can self-advocate. One way to advocate for yourself is to show the prepared materials you brought with you to the doctor. By providing the symptom and medication lists to the provider, you are showing yourself to be actively involved in your diagnosis and care. While the doctor is making their clinical assessment, there may be things discussed that you may not understand. Ask questions and keep asking questions until you understand. Here is a list of some general questions you may want to ask.

- Can you explain the diagnosis to me in layman's terms?
- What does _____ mean?
- What causes this disease/condition?
- Can you explain why you are recommending this diagnostic test and what it checks?

- Are there any drawbacks or side effects to the tests you are recommending?
- Is there anything else that could be causing my symptoms?
- Can you repeat the next steps?
- Am I contagious? Can I pass this on to my family members? If so, what precautions should I take?
- How does this diagnosis affect my body?
- What are the expectations for this diagnosis? How long will it take for me to get better?
- How are the treatments tolerated by those with the same diagnosis?
- How will the medication you are prescribing help treat the condition?
- Will the new medications you are prescribing interact with the ones I am currently taking?
- Are there any alternative treatments for this diagnosis?
- Will lifestyle changes help me heal from this diagnosis?
- Are there any risks to the treatments?
- Is there a symptom I might have that may indicate my condition is getting worse?

- How will this diagnosis affect my home and work life?
- Will I need a follow-up visit? Can we extend the time of my appointment if we need more time for questions?
- Do you have any reading materials I can take with me and share with my family about this diagnosis?
- Can you please recap my next steps?

For more specific diagnoses, such as cancer, please refer to the References & Resources section for questions to ask your medical provider.

You may find that you have more questions after the visit has ended. Usually, there is a way to submit your questions through a web-based portal if your medical office uses one. The questions are usually routed to the nursing staff, who can then send them to the doctor if they cannot answer them.

Asking questions during your medical visit will alleviate your anxiety, communicate to your doctor that you are concerned and motivated to learn more about your diagnosis, and show active participation and advocacy for your health. Now that you have more information from your doctor, who serves as your trusted source, you can conduct research on your own via the internet. Remember to only use trusted websites to do your research (refer to Chapter 2 for reputable and trusted websites).

You may find more information about alternative treatments, information on recommended diagnostic tests, and determine other questions you may want to ask your doctor at your follow-up visit. The more curious you are about your disease/condition, the more questions you will generate. Be curious, speak up for yourself, use direct eye contact with the doctor, place your phone or device on silent, pay close attention, and remain engaged. It may be difficult to do all these things based on the information you receive, but try hard to stay engaged. If it was challenging to stay engaged and focused during the initial medical visit, consider bringing someone with you to the follow-up visit. Make sure the person you bring is someone you trust, can remain engaged, is curious, and can advocate for you in the event you cannot.

After the initial medical visit, evaluate how you think the visit went. Did you feel like your questions were answered to your satisfaction? Did you understand the information that was shared? Did you feel like you expressed your concerns well? What would you do differently for the next visit? Do you need to bring someone with you next time for emotional support? Did the doctor recognize your advocacy and your participation in your own health?

If there is no follow-up or this was your first time approaching a medical visit in this manner, celebrate your win. Many people don't ask questions and are passive participants in their medical appointments, but you're not one of them! You made a choice to approach this differently, and it could change the course of your disease/condition for the better. It is perfectly fine to form a trusting relationship with your doctor or healthcare team. You are part of this team, too. Honesty is what makes this team effective because that is the only way the treatment plan can work. Asking questions and negotiating your preferences will help the team be more successful. For example, if the treatment plan includes you performing certain tasks in the morning and you are not a morning person, communicate that to the team and determine if these steps can be done later in the day and still be effective. If you are prescribed pills as a treatment and you have trouble swallowing pills, ask if a different form of the medication can be prescribed to you based on your preference. **Bottom line: you are as important to this team as the doctor. If you are unable to perform what the doctor is prescribing, then you will not be able to improve your health condition.**

It is an ultimate hope that you can form a trusting relationship with your medical provider. This is the best-case scenario, as you want to feel like the healthcare team is on the same page concerning your health. However, sometimes this trusting relationship does not exist. You may feel like you are not on the same page with the treatment plan, you may not feel respected, or you just don't feel the connection.

Research from Yale University shows that some people feel more comfortable with a medical provider who is of the same gender. Additionally, a recent study also showed that people belonging to racial/ethnic minority groups who share the same race/ethnicity as the medical provider have improved communication, better perceptions of care, and better health outcomes.[12] The study also showed that patients who did not have a preference for race/ethnicity emphasized professionalism over race, valued diverse perspectives, and appreciated their providers' cultural awareness and willingness to self-educate.

Ultimately, if you feel the lack of a genuine connection with your medical provider may impede your progress, you should switch to a provider where you have the connection you desire. Your health is paramount, and finding a better team player could be necessary for your success. There are many great doctors who may better align with your needs.

---

[12] Moore et al., 2022

# After the Medical Visit

After the medical visit, try not to feel overwhelmed with the information you have gathered about your disease/condition. If you took notes, make sure you understand all the information that was shared and the next steps that were discussed.

If you were given handouts, make sure you have read them and shared them with your loved ones, if you choose. Were there things you discussed that you can do on your own to positively affect your medical diagnosis? How many things did you discuss? If it was a list of items, start off with one at a time. If it helps, start with the easiest one to incorporate into your daily routine. By many accounts, it can take twenty-one days to form a new habit. Give yourself at least three weeks to adjust to the first change you make. (If you need a strategy or plan to adopt a new habit or behavior, please refer to the References & Resources section in the back of this book for a link to the worksheet on creating a new habit.)

Once you feel like you have established a routine with one change, then move to the second suggestion on the list. Keep going with this rhythm until you have incorporated all or most of the suggestions into your daily activities. You might find that you are having trouble incorporating some of the suggestions mentioned during the medical visit. If so, discuss whether the suggestion is necessary at your follow-up visit, considering the other changes you have made. Discuss what you have been doing and ask for ideas on how you can achieve this step toward your health journey.

You may have been given new medications to treat your diagnosis. You may not have ever taken these medications before, and you want to be sure to listen to your body (refer to Step 1) to determine how well you are adjusting to the new medication. If you are not reacting well to the medication, be sure to write down the symptoms you are experiencing. It may be helpful to use the symptom list we discussed in Step 3. Before contacting the medical professional, be sure you read the side effects information provided by the pharmacy to determine if what you are experiencing is expected or typical. You will want to let the doctor know via their preferred mode of communication (phone call, email, or messaging via their web-based portal) if your symptoms worsen.

It is not recommended that you stop taking medication without alerting the doctor. Some medications require you to taper off instead of abruptly stopping. Effective communication during this process is key so you can continue improving on your health journey. Resolving issues quickly is the best way to achieve that goal.

# Advocating for Family Members

Over the course of this book, we have learned steps to advocate for ourselves during the medical visit. These steps are vital for your care and the care of others you love. There are many family members who are caregivers, whether it is to family members with physical/mental disabilities or to those who are aging. According to the World Health Organization, "the population aged 60 years and over will increase from 1 billion in 2020 to 1.4 billion. By 2050, the world's population of people aged 60 years and older will double (2.1 billion). The number of persons aged 80 years or older is expected to triple between 2020 and 2050 to reach 426 million."

Many people, as they age, require caregivers to assist them in their lives. Caregivers provide care, support, and assistance to someone who needs help with daily activities or has a chronic illness. Caregivers are also in a perfect position to advocate for those family members during medical visits, due to their natural proximity to the patient.

Many of the same steps outlined in this book can be followed by the caregiver to advocate for family members during medical visits. However, one very important starting point is to make sure the trust between the caregiver and the family member is secure and that they have your best interest at the forefront before moving forward with advocacy. The goal is always to obtain the best care for the patient. It is not about the caregiver and his/her needs (that is a separate issue that is very important to address). Be sure the family member is comfortable with you speaking for them, with you helping them make decisions regarding their care, and that you can be emotionally supportive of them.

Another thing caregivers should be aware of is Medicare benefits. Wikipedia defines Medicare as "a federal health insurance program in the United States for people age 65 or older and younger people with disabilities." There are different benefit options, and they can include out-of-pocket costs for Medicare coverage. Families must be educated on this program and which option best suits the family member's needs now and for the future.

The steps of advocacy outlined in previous chapters are also appropriate for those patients with caregivers, with minor changes. For example, for Step 1, the caregiver must inquire with the family member regarding symptoms. The caregiver may have to ask a series of questions and complete the symptom diary on the patient's behalf to prepare for the medical visit. The caregiver must be able to communicate with the family member well enough to gather helpful information about the condition, which can then be communicated to the medical professional so the patient can receive optimal care. Being aware of family history, having a list of medications and dosages, and encouraging honesty about the health history are best whether you are the patient or the caregiver (Steps 2-3).

One addition to Step 4 is to make sure the family member is able to ask questions, if they choose to. We always want to respect their voice and opinion at every stage, even though they have entrusted you with their care and to make decisions on their behalf. Remember, the patient is a valuable part of the healthcare team and must see themselves that way. If you are the caregiver, you must speak for the family member with one voice and in the way they would for themselves.

Lastly, the final step in advocacy is reviewing the materials from the visit and making sure you and the patient understand what was communicated about the disease/condition (Step 5). Make sure to use reputable websites to educate yourselves further about the diagnosis and continue to make a list of questions for the follow-up visit. If medication was prescribed, make sure to be observant and ask questions to determine if there are any side effects that need to be communicated to the medical team.

Many of the advocacy steps are the same, whether you are advocating for yourself or someone else. However, extra care is needed to advocate for someone who has entrusted you with this task. Make sure they have a voice at every step and you have their best interest at the forefront as they proceed through their healthcare journey.

# Action Plan: You Got This!

Now that you have the steps to start advocating for yourself, it is time to put them into practice. The most important thing to remember is that you, your thoughts, and your questions are just as important during a medical visit as the doctor's diagnosis and treatment plan. Your participation, buy-in, and clear understanding are crucial in performing the recommendations offered to assist in your healing. You must show up as your authentic self, be calm, and be able to focus so that you can impact your health for the better.

Remember that your ability to stay calm and focus is vital, as you may not know if the information you receive as a diagnosis will be good news or bad news. Throughout your lifetime, you may have been in several situations where you have received bad news. As you recall those times, how did you react? Were you able to think clearly and make good decisions considering the news? If you have been unsuccessful in those moments, consider taking a trusted person with you to the visit and/or the follow-up visit. This person will be able to ask questions, take notes, and listen carefully on your behalf.

**Bottom line: It is very important in your advocacy role to understand the information shared with you so you can act on it to improve your health. You Got This!**

Remember the steps:

- You are a very important part of the medical visit. Show up, advocate, and be empowered!
- Listen to your body and pay attention to what it is telling you.
- Know your Family Health History—you can't change your family history, but you can increase the chances of prevention with what you learn. Knowledge is power.
- Prepare for the medical visit by bringing your symptom diary, list of your medications (including vitamins and supplements), and being open and honest with the provider.

- Ask questions and listen carefully for the answers. If you don't understand something, ask additional questions.
- Ask for reading materials about the diagnosis you received to review at home.
- When you get back home, think about what happened during the visit. Reflect on what went well and any additional questions you would like to ask during a follow-up visit. If you choose, talk to your loved ones about what you learned about your health.
- If new medications were prescribed, listen closely to your body again. Keep a new symptom diary for your next appointment, if necessary.
- Don't stop medications abruptly. Consult your doctor before stopping a new medication.
- Use trusted websites to conduct further research on your diagnosis, like NIH and CDC.

Your advocacy on your health journey can change your health trajectory for the better. As you grow in your own advocacy, you can begin to reach out to family members, teach them the skills you have learned, and/or advocate for others in their healthcare situation. The knowledge you gain will continue to grow and reach others, potentially aiding in the reduction of health disparities in specific communities. As more people adopt this philosophy, imagine how many health trajectories can change. In our lifetime, we can change how the data shows higher occurrences of chronic diseases among specific populations. Future research studies investigating how self-advocacy can affect health disparities among specific communities have yet to be studied and published. I am excited to see this research in the future, but I am even more excited to see increased empowerment levels in all communities, especially among African Americans and Hispanics. You Got This!

"Change will not come if we wait for some other person or some other time. We are the ones we have been waiting for. We are the change that we seek."

—Barack Obama

# Acknowledgments and Gratitude

**God** - Heavenly Father, this idea and book would not exist without you. It came to be at a time of upheaval and uncertainty in my life. Once I decided this was where I could be productive and bring to life a long-held dream, *you* allowed the words to rapidly flow. I am eternally grateful to you for ordering my steps and pointing me in this direction. I also thank you for planting the idea in my head almost twenty years ago as I started my career in public health. I pray that readers will think differently about interacting in the healthcare space after reading these words. Ultimately, I pray that readers become more empowered and advocate for themselves in healthcare spaces, as well as in every other aspect of life. Amen.

**My family and friends** – I am grateful for your love. You have been so supportive and encouraging of this dream. Thank you for always believing in me and thinking I can do anything I set my mind to, and it will be done with excellence. Thank you for providing me with the space I needed to create, think, and produce. Hailey, thank you for brainstorming this idea with me in North Carolina. I will never forget how excited you were to help me bring this dream to life. Alex, thank you for being so supportive in your own way. Thank you for encouraging me all the way from Syracuse, NY. Kacy, thank you for being so excited when I told you this was my new project. Thank you for doing everything you could to find me a tool to create this book. Mom and Dad, thank you for always being you—so supportive in every way. Thank you for your encouraging words and for the ways you always offer to support me. I am truly grateful to have such wonderful parents. Reg, thank you for our thought-provoking conversations around this book. Our conversations helped me shape the content of some chapters, and I am so grateful to and for you. Tanya, thank you for your eagle eye and for helping me transform my writing from scholarly to something more understandable to many. Juan, thank you for supporting me through a tumultuous time and showing excitement about this idea and all my progress. Thank you for always helping me look at things from a different perspective and being willing to support me always.

Thank you to all my awesome and wonderful friends. When I told you about this project, each of you was extremely supportive. You asked questions, followed up, and told me you were proud of my resilience. I appreciate each of you and thank you from the bottom of my heart.

**Stefanie Taylor** – I want to sincerely thank you for the idea to write this book. The idea was one that was born during my career as a federal employee. I don't even remember talking about this idea with you when we were neighbors, but you did. That was several years ago. However, the notion that it could come to life as a book came from you on February 25, 2025. For that, I am eternally grateful. Your friendship at that moment showed me that it is important to have people around you that think differently than you, who have a vision for your life, and believe in you.

# References & Resources

## PREFACE

Healthy People 2020.
https://www.cdc.gov/nchs/healthy_people/hp2020.htm.

## THE SCIENCE

Collier AY and Molina RL. Maternal mortality in the United States: Updates on trends, causes, and solutions. Neoreviews. 2019 October: 20 (10): e561-e574.

The White House. The White House Blueprint for Addressing the Maternal Health Crisis: Two Years of Progress (2024). https://bidenwhitehouse.archives.gov/briefing-room/statements-releases/2024/07/10/the-white-house-blueprint-for-addressing-the-maternal-health-crisis-two-years-of-progress/.

Mayo Clinic. What is a Stroke? https://www.mayoclinic.org/diseases-conditions/stroke/symptoms-causes/syc-20350113.

Centers for Disease Control and Prevention (CDC). Stroke: Stroke facts. https://www.cdc.gov/stroke/data-research/facts-stats/.

Diaz JA, Griffith RA, NG JJ, Reinert SE, Friedmann PD and Moulton AW. Patients' use of the internet for medical information. Journal of General Internal Medicine. 2002; 17; 180-185.

Wang X and Cohen RA. Health information technology use among adults: United States, July-December 2022. 2023 October; National Center for Health Statistics (NCHS) Data Brief (482).

National Institutes of Health (NIH). Accessed at www.nih.gov.

U.S. Office of Personnel Management (OPM): Plain Language. https://www.opm.gov/information-management/plain-language/.

## THE GOAL OF ADVOCACY

Weill Cornell Medicine. Empowering teens to be their own health advocates, 2021, https://weillcornell.org/news/empowering-teens-to-be-their-own-health-advocates.

## STEP 1: LISTEN TO YOUR BODY

Hodge B. The use of symptom diaries in outpatient care, May/June 2013, www.aafp.org/fpm.

Centers for Disease Control and Prevention (CDC), Sleep, https://www.cdc.gov/sleep/about/index.html.

## STEP 2: KNOW YOUR FAMILY HEALTH HISTORY

US Surgeon General. My Family Health Portrait. https://cbiit.github.io/FHH/html/index.html.

Hull LE. and Natarajan P. Self-rated family health history knowledge among *All of Us* program participants. Genet Med. 2022 April 24(4): 955-961.

The "Does It Run in the Family?" tool gives the 'why' and 'how' behind collecting family health history information, tips for talking to family members, examples of conditions that can run in the family, and hints for health. It is customizable with personal health stories, photos, and health condition information. https://doesitruninthefamily.org

National Institutes of Health - National Heart, Lung, and Blood Institute. Family History and High Blood Pressure - Family History Worksheet. https://www.nia.nih.gov/sites/default/files/2021-06/worksheet-family-health-history.pdf

## STEP 3: PREPARE FOR THE MEDICAL VISIT

Healthwise. Diary of Symptoms
https://content.healthwise.net/resources/14.3/en-us/media/pdf/hw/form_tm6566.pdf

National Institutes of Health - National Institute on Aging. Medication Worksheet.
https://www.nia.nih.gov/sites/default/files/2023-05/twyd-medications-worksheet.pdf

## STEP 4: SPEAK UP AND ASK QUESTIONS AT THE MEDICAL VISIT AND BEYOND

Smith-Slade. Addiction Center. 2025. Why it is important to be honest about substance use with your doctor.
https://www.addictioncenter.com/community/honest-substance-use-doctor/.

Moore C., Coates E., Watson A., de Heer R., McLeod A., and Prudhomme A. "It's important to work with people that look like me": Black patients' preferences for patient-provider race concordance. Journal of Racial and Ethnic Health Disparities. 2022. https://doi.org/10.1007/s40615-022-01435-y

National Institutes of Health: National Institute on Aging. Changes to Discuss.

https://www.nia.nih.gov/sites/default/files/2021-06/worksheet-changes-to-discuss.pdf

National Institutes of Health: National Institute on Aging. Concerns. https://www.nia.nih.gov/sites/default/files/2021-06/worksheet-concerns.pdf

American Cancer Society. Questions to ask about your Cancer. https://www.cancer.org/cancer/managing-cancer/making-treatment-decisions/questions-to-ask-about-treatment.html

## ADVOCATING FOR FAMILY MEMBERS

World Health Organization. Ageing and Health. 2025. https://www.who.int/news-room/fact-sheets/detail/ageing-and-health

## ACTION PLAN

Grand Valley State University: University Counseling Center. Creating New Habits. https://www.gvsu.edu/cms4/asset/8BE68CB1-B1E8-CE01-5CD0C1D211317763/creating_new_habits_worksheet.pdf

# About the Author

**HENRAYA MCGRUDER, PHD** is a former senior research scientist in the Office on Smoking and Health, Centers for Disease Control and Prevention, and a retired Lieutenant Commander in the United States Public Health Services. During her twenty-two-year career, she has served in many roles, from Epidemiologist to Public Health Advisor, across various divisions at CDC. Dr. McGruder began her career at CDC in 2002 as an Epidemic Intelligence Service officer, where she was assigned to the Cardiovascular Health Branch. She is a subject matter expert in emergency response, tobacco cessation, and health disparities among persons with chronic diseases. She has published several scholarly articles in scientific journals, including Stroke, Ethnicity & Disease, Preventing Chronic Disease, Morbidity & Mortality Weekly Report (MMWR), among others. In 2022, Henraya founded Audacious Health Advocates, LLC, to help individuals understand the value and importance of advocating for their own health. This organization is an outgrowth of her research on health disparities and her need to find ways to eliminate them in various populations. Dr. McGruder also has over a decade of teaching experience as a professor of psychology, serving at Spelman College and Johnson C. Smith University.

Dr. McGruder is a native of Atlanta, Georgia. She holds a bachelor's degree in psychology from Hampton University and master's and Ph.D. in neuropsychology from Howard University. In her free time, she enjoys spending time with her family, traveling, and listening to live music. She is the mother of two children, Alexander and Hailey, and the wife of Juan A. McGruder, PhD.